Book 1:
Thyroid Diet
BY LINDSEY P

&

Book 2:
The Hypothyroidism Handbook
BY LINDSEY P

Book 1:
Thyroid Diet
BY LINDSEY P

Easy Guide to Managing Thyroid Symptoms, Losing Weight, Increasing Your Metabolism

ESSENTIAL OILS BOX SET #16: Thyroid Diet & The Hypothyroidism Handbook

Copyright 2014 by Lindsey P - All rights reserved.

In no way is it legal to reproduce, duplicate, or transmit any part of this document in either electronic means or in printed format. Recording of this publication is strictly prohibited and any storage of this document is not allowed unless with written permission from the publisher. All rights reserved.

ESSENTIAL OILS BOX SET #16: Thyroid Diet & The Hypothyroidism Handbook

Table Of Contents

Introduction 5
Chapter 1   **Your Thyroid** 6
Chapter 2   **Thyroid Imbalances** 8
Chapter 3   **Restoring Balance Through Diet** 12
Chapter 4   **Thyroid Diet** 15
Chapter 5   **Thyroid Diet Food Guide** 19
Chapter 6   **Thyroid Diet for Weight Loss** 24
Conclusion 25

ESSENTIAL OILS BOX SET #16: Thyroid Diet & The Hypothyroidism Handbook

Introduction

I want to thank you and congratulate you for purchasing the book, *"Thyroid Diet: Easy Guide To Managing Thyroid Symptoms, Losing Weight, Increasing Your Metabolism"*

This book contains proven steps and strategies on how to take care of your thyroid gland. This small gland located in the neck drives the body's metabolism. Imbalance of the hormonal functions would mean disturbances in different aspects of the body, like digestion, weight control and energy. Even sleep can get affected, too.

In this book, learn all about the thyroid gland, its hormones, its functions and how you can keep it healthy. A healthy organ is a healthy body. Learn about how the thyroid function can go off balance. Know about the different disorders related to it, the causes and how these can be managed.

Also, learn about the thyroid diet- what is it, what can it do and how you can use it for yourself. There are a lot of things you need to learn about your body. Start with your thyroid.

Thanks again for purchasing this book, I hope you enjoy it!

Chapter 1 Your Thyroid

Each and every organ in the body, big or small, plays an important role in the body. Each function is an integral part of a whole complex of chemical and metabolic processes that keep the body in homeostasis. One of the small organs with huge important function is the thyroid gland.

Located in front of the neck, the thyroid gland sits just below the Adam's apple and in front of the windpipe. It has a butterfly shape, each "wing" is a lobe connected to each other via an isthmus located between them. This gland is normally brownish red from the rich blood supply from its abundant blood vessels.

The thyroid gland is about 2 inches big. It is composed of 2 cell types, namely, the follicular and the parafollicular cells. The follicular cells make up most of the thyroid tissues. These cells are responsible in secreting the hormones thyroxine (T4) and triiodothyronine (T3). On the other hand, parafollicular cells are responsible for the secretion of another thyroid hormone called calcitonin.

Thyroid Gland Function

The main function of the thyroid gland is to regulate the metabolism and calcium balance in the body. This function is carried out by the various thyroid hormones. The T3 and T4 hormones regulate metabolism. Calcitonin helps in maintaining calcium balance.

The signal to start and stop thyroid hormone synthesis and secretion comes from the thyroid-stimulating hormone secreted by the pituitary gland. The hypothalamus, in turn, sends a signal to the pituitary gland to regulate the signaling mechanism.

Thyroid Hormones

Three basic thyroid hormones work with the rest of the body in order to maintain homeostasis. These hormones are T3, T4 and calcitonin. T4 and T3 are considered as the main thyroid hormones, as they carry out the

T4 and T3 hormones are produced by the follicular cells of the thyroid gland. Iodine plays an important role in the production of these 2 hormones.

T3 and T4 stimulate the various cells in the body. They promote protein synthesis and increase the rate of cellular oxygen consumption. In absence of these hormones, the body cannot breakdown and metabolizes proteins, vitamins and carbohydrates.

T3 and T4 work together to influence other endocrine glands, as well. They influence the production and release of adrenaline and epinephrine. T3 and T4 also play a role in dopamine production and secretion in the brain.

The thyroid makes sure that there is adequate, steady and ready supply of T3 and T4 in the body. A few "droplets" of these hormones are stored within the thyroid gland, ready for release once TSH (thyroid stimulating hormone) sends a signal for their release and activation. Some of T3 and T4 are bound to carrier proteins and circulate in the blood. This is why blood tests can reveal if there are sufficient thyroid hormones in the body.

If the body needs thyroid hormones at any given time, the carrier proteins free the bound T3 and T4 hormones. These hormones would then travel to the cells that need them and work their effect.

Together, T3 and T4 increase the body's basal metabolic rate. That would mean the following bodily responses:

- Rise in body temperature
- Stronger heartbeat
- increased pulse
- Faster digestion and use of ingested food
- Faster utilization of energy resources stored in the muscles and liver
- Promotes brain maturation in children
- Growth promotion in children
- Activation of the nervous system, causing better levels of attention and Better reflex action

Calcitonin hormone plays a role in maintaining calcium balance in the body. It works together with hormones produced by another gland called the parathyroid glands. The C-cells within the thyroid gland synthesize this hormone. It plays vital roles in calcium regulation and bone metabolism.

Chapter 2 Thyroid Imbalance

Thyroid gland function can become compromised, leading to inadequate circulating and stored hormones. Imbalances in thyroid hormone production can affect all aspects of body function, which includes weight regulation, control and regulation of other hormones, digestion process, live function, and a whole lot more.

Causes of Thyroid Problems

There are basically two types of thyroid imbalance- hyper and hypo. Hyperthyroidism means the thyroid gland is producing more hormones than necessary. Hypothyroidism means the thyroid gland is not producing adequate amounts of hormones.

Hyperthyroidism is caused by the following:

- Graves' disease

  This is a result of overproduction of thyroid hormones.

- Toxic adenomas

  Sometimes, nodules grow in the thyroid. These nodules can secrete thyroid hormones that can upset the hormonal balance. Some goiters have nodules that have hormone-secreting capacity.

- Subacute thyroiditis

  This is an inflammatory condition of the thyroid gland. The inflammation causes the stored thyroid hormones to leak out of the gland and into the blood. This will cause an increase in the amounts of circulating thyroid hormones, leading to hyperthyroidism. In this case, hyperthyroidism may be temporary, lasting for a few weeks to a few months. Generally, the hormonal imbalance will resolve on its own after the thyroid gland inflammation subsides.

- Malfunctioning pituitary gland

  The pituitary gland sends the signal for thyroid hormone production. More pituitary gland signaling means more thyroid hormone production. Sometimes, tumors and other pituitary problems can cause more signals sent for thyroid hormone synthesis leading to hyperthyroidism.

Hypothyroidism is too little production of thyroid hormones. This would cause too little energy for metabolic processes. Common causes of hypothyroidism include:

- Hashimoto's thyroiditis

    This is an autoimmune disease attacks and destroys the cells in the thyroid glands. The thyroid cells eventually die, causing the gland to produce less hormones.

- Thyroid gland removal

    Destruction and removal of the thyroid gland may cause inadequate hormone production. This may be due to surgical removal or chemical destruction.

- Excessive exposure to iodide

    Hypothyroidism may also be caused by too much exposure to iodine. This may come from use of contrast dyes, sinus and cold medicines, and cardiac medicines such as amiodarone.

- Lithium

    In some individuals, taking lithium has been found to cause a decrease in the circulating thyroid hormones.

Signs and Symptoms of Thyroid Problems

Thyroid problems may manifest in a wide range of symptoms. The most common ones are the following:

- Fatigue

    This is the most common symptom of thyroid problems. It may be vague but it is the most commonly experienced symptom. A person wakes up feeling tired despite getting adequate amounts if sleep. All throughout the day, the need to nap is very common. Also, people with hyperthyroidism have difficulty falling asleep or maintaining a restful sleep.

- Weight changes

    Weight is heavily influenced by thyroid hormones. Often, difficulty losing weight despite low-fat and calorie diets coupled with rigorous exercise is a sign of hypothyroidism. Unintentional weight loss despite no changes in the amount of consumed food is a sign of hyperthyroidism.

- Heat intolerance

    People with hyperthyroidism would often feel warmer than usual.

- Feels cold easily

    Hypothyroidism causes a person to feel cold all the time, with no relation at all to weather or room temperature.

- Pain in the muscles and joints

    Thyroid hormones influence calcium and energy consumption by the bones and muscles. Often, thyroid problems can cause muscle and joint aches and pains. It may also cause weakness in the muscles and joints that can further develop into carpal tunnel syndrome (in the hands or arms), tarsal tunnel syndrome (in the legs) and plantar fasciitis in the feet.

- Discomfort or enlargement of the neck

    Thyroid enlargement may cause outward signs such as swelling or enlargement in the neck area. It may also be manifested as discomfort when wearing something over the neck such as scarves and neckties.

- Changes in the hair and/or skin

    The hair and the skin are sensitive to changes in the thyroid function. Hypothyroidism would often cause the hair to become dry, coarse, and brittle breaks off and falls easily. It can also cause the outer edge of the eyebrows to fall off. The skin becomes dry, thick, scaly and coarse.

    Hyperthyroidism can cause severe hair loss. The skin becomes thin and fragile, causing it to become injured easily.

- Changes in the bowel function

    Thyroid hormones influence other systems as well. Problems in the thyroid function can also cause changes in the functioning of other systems. In the digestive system, hypothyroidism can cause severe or chronic constipation. Hyperthyroidism can cause IBS (irritable bowel syndrome) or frequent diarrhea.

- Reproductive changes

    Women who have thyroid problems often experience irregularities in their menstrual periods. Hyperthyroidism is often associated with infrequent periods. Menstruation is often of short duration with lighter flow. Hypothyroidism causes menstrual periods to occur more often. Flow is often heavier and more painful.

    Fertility is also affected by thyroid imbalance. There may be infertility concerns in both men and women.

- Cholesterol problems

    High cholesterol levels unresponsive to diet, medication and exercise are often associated with hypothyroidism. Very low cholesterol that is unusual may be signifying hyperthyroidism.

- Mental changes

  Hypothyroidism is often associated with depression. Hyperthyroidism is associated with panic or anxiety attacks.

- Tremors and nervousness

  Hyperthyroidism causes muscle tremors, agitation and nervousness.

- Bloated

  From fluid retention due to hypothyroidism

- Tachycardia and palpitations

Chapter 3 Restoring Balance through Diet

Nutrition plays an important role in regulating thyroid function. A lot of nutrients can increase or decrease this gland's function. Some improve the cell susceptibility to thyroid hormones. Some are used as part of the hormone synthesis process.

Iodine

This is the single most important nutrient for thyroid health. The hormones T3 and T4 rely on the presence of iodine for production. One of the main causes of thyroid dysfunction is due to iodine deficiency.

The body has no capacity to manufacture this trace element. It needs to be obtained from dietary sources. Iodine from food is released through the digestive process. It is then absorbed by the intestines and brought to the blood stream. The blood then brings iodine to the thyroid glands, where it becomes part of thyroid hormone production.

Major source of iodine is iodized salt. This fortified salt ensures that people will be getting the recommended daily amounts of this very important trace mineral. Other sources include grains, fish and dairy.

Iodine supplements are one of the options for treating deficiencies and improving thyroid function. However, excess iodine can cause thyroid imbalance and other problems, too. People with Hashimoto's disease may experience flare-ups with iodine supplements.

Vitamin D

A study showed that Hashimoto's disease and vitamin D deficiency are linked. About 90% of patients with this form of thyroid disorder have been found to be deficient in vitamin D.

Patients with Grave's disease also suffer from bone loss. Vitamin D worsens bone loss in this disorder. The loss of bone mass often resolves as thyroid condition improves. Experts agree that it can also be treated by giving vitamin D supplements, especially before and after thyroid treatments.

Food sources rich in vitamin D include milk, dairy, eggs, mushrooms and fatty fish. Supplemental vitamin D3 is also given to some patients. While on supplemental D3, the patient needs to be constantly monitored to ensure that the vitamin D levels should be within the desired therapeutic range.

Selenium

Selenium in the body is concentrated in the thyroid gland. This mineral is a component of important enzymes that influence thyroid function. Also, it has

ESSENTIAL OILS BOX SET #16: Thyroid Diet & The Hypothyroidism Handbook

been found that selenium can affect cognitive function, immune system, mortality and fertility in both men and women.

Studies have found that selenium boosts the levels of circulating thyroid hormones. It also improves the mood of people suffering from Hashimoto's disease.

On the other hand, excessive selenium intake can cause health problems such as gastrointestinal upset. Too much selenium can also increase the risk for type 2 diabetes and some cancers.

Selenium levels should be constantly monitored while on supplements and treatment. Selenium-rich foods are less likely to cause serious side effects. Good food sources include tuna, Brazil nuts, lobster and crabs.

Vitamin B12

Studies made among people with thyroid disorders have found that about 30% also suffer from vitamin B12 deficiency. Severe deficiency with this vitamin is irreversible and having a thyroid disorder can worsen the problem. Supplement with food sources like seafood such as salmon, sardines and mollusks. Other great sources of vitamin B12 include dairy, lean meats and organ meats such as the liver. Plant sources of vitamin B12 include nutritional yeast and fortified cereals.

Goitrogens

Goitrogens are foods that have been found to interfere with thyroid hormone synthesis. The active compound in these foods is called goitrin. This compound is released when the food is hydrolyzed. However, goitrin only becomes a concern if there is an existing iodine deficiency state in the body. Also, goitrin is easily denatured (destroyed or inactivated) and the goitrogenic effects rendered ineffective when is heated. Well-known goitrogenic foods are the cruciferous vegetables like cauliflower, cabbage and broccoli.

Aside from cruciferous vegetables, soy is also a potential goitrogen. Soy contains the compounds isoflavones, which can slow down the rate of thyroid hormone synthesis. However, soy does not directly cause hypothyroidism. The isoflavones do not cause profound thyroid imbalance if there are good iodine stores in the body.

Millet is another potential goitrogen. This gluten-free, nutritious grain has been found to affect thyroid function. People with adequate iodine stores experience suppression of their thyroid function when consuming millet. People suffering from hypothyroidism are especially advised to avoid taking millet.

Medications and Supplements

Some medications and supplements have been found to affect thyroid function. Calcium supplements may help with reducing bone loss, but can interfere with the absorption of thyroid medications. In order to harness the benefits of calcium supplements and reduce the interference with thyroid medications, patients are advised to take these separately. Experts advise waiting at least 4 hours in between taking calcium supplements and thyroid medications.

Fiber supplements and coffee have also been found to lower the rate of absorption of thyroid medication. In order to decrease the interference from these foods, take them at least 1 hour apart.

Another compound that interferes with thyroid function and thyroid medication is chromium picolinate. This compound is marketed for weight loss and blood sugar control. Taking chromium picolinate lowers thyroid hormone function and interferes with thyroid medication action. Take them at least 3 to 4 hours apart.

Fruits, green tea and vegetables contain beneficial flavonoids that have great health benefits. They improve cardiovascular health and helps in preventing several serious illnesses like stroke and cancers. However, studies have shown that taking large amounts of flavonoids, especially in supplemental forms, suppress the action of thyroid hormones. Experts recommend consulting a dietician and physician in order to get a balance of flavonoid benefits and thyroid function.

ESSENTIAL OILS BOX SET #16: Thyroid Diet & The Hypothyroidism Handbook

Chapter 4 Thyroid Diet

In order to help return the balance and normal function of the thyroid gland, experts have formulated the thyroid diet. The aim of this diet is to

Thyroid diet is an individualized diet that aims to provide the necessary nutrients the body needs while improving thyroid function. To start, calculate the calories needed by the body on a daily basis. Then make adjustments depending on the desired outcome of the thyroid diet.

Calories

To get the daily caloric needs:

1. Get the current body weight in kilograms. If using pounds, convert the weight to kilograms by dividing the value by 2.2.

   Thus, for a person weighing 165 pounds, convert it to kilograms by dividing it by 2.2, which will yield 75 kilograms.

2. Multiply the weight (in kilograms) by 30. The number 30 refers to the number of calories the body needs for each pound of body weight.

   For the same person above, multiply the weight of 75 kilograms by 30, which is 2250. So, theoretically, a person weighing 75 kilograms needs 2250 calories in a day.

3. From the computed daily calorie needs, subtract 200. This is an estimation that reflects the need to reduce the calorie intake in relation to the thyroid condition.

   Therefore, a person who weighs 75 kilograms needs 2250 calories in a day. Because of a thyroid condition, less calories is needed in order to maintain the same 75-kilogram weight. Hence, in order to maintain the current weight, the person with a thyroid condition needs 2050 calories in a day.

4. If the goal of going on a thyroid diet is to lose weight, the daily calorie requirements should be reduced by 5 calories for each kilogram of body weight. That would be multiplying the weight in kilograms by 25 instead of 30.

   So, a person who weighs 75 kilograms and wants to lose weight using the thyroid diet would multiply the weight by 25 instead of 30. That will be 1875 calories per day. This, in theory, is the daily calorie need in order to lose 1 pound of body weight every 10 days.

Then subtract the 200 calories to account for the thyroid condition. Thus, a person weighing 75 kilograms who has a thyroid condition and wants to use the thyroid diet for weight loss would need to take 1675 calories per day in order to lose weight safely.

Pillars of the Thyroid Diet

The thyroid diet is formulated based on the following basic concepts:

I. Protecting the thyroid from harmful substances

Most thyroid imbalances are caused by the destruction or damage to the thyroid gland. Inflammation causes hormones to leak out into the blood, cellular destruction can cause low hormone production. Remove substances that are detrimental to thyroid health.

   a. Sugar

   Fluctuations in the sugar levels can cause hormones to go off balance, including the thyroid hormones. If there is sugar imbalance in the body, thyroid function will a take a long time to improve. This is because the pancreas that regulates sugar metabolism also affects thyroid function.

   Limit daily sugar intake to no more than 5 spoons. In 1 teaspoon of sugar, there are 4 grams of sugar. In a tablespoon, 12 grams of sugar is present.

   Combat sugar cravings by eating a high protein, high fat breakfast. Energy from these foods will help tide the body over until lunch, which completely avoids the mid-morning energy and sugar crash that leads to cravings.

   b. Food Intolerances

   Most people experience thyroid disturbances when eating gluten-containing foods. Eliminating it from the diet has shown improvement in their thyroid conditions. Also, it may be necessary to eliminate more than gluten it usually needs to eliminate the big 5- foods that are common causes of food intolerances. The big 5 are gluten, soy, dairy, eggs and corn.

   c. Improve gut health

   The gut or the digestive system plays an important role in managing thyroid disorders. A huge concentration of immune cells such as lymphocytes is present in the gut. Imbalance in this part would often cause autoimmune disorders, one of the leading causes of thyroid dysfunction.

d. Avoid toxic substances

Avoid foods that contain toxic ingredients such as preservatives, additives, excessive sodium, artificial sweeteners and trans fats. Also, avoid exposure to environmental toxins from house cleaners and other substances.

Water toxicity has been found to be an increasing contributing factor to thyroid problems. Fluoride in water has been linked to hypothyroidism. This element has been found to enter the thyroid gland and reduce iodine uptake. Decreased uptake of iodine means slowed production of T4 thyroid hormone.

e. Detoxify

T4 hormone is inactive and needs to be converted into active T3 in order to work its effects on the body. Conversion happens in the liver and the digestive tract. Sluggish liver and gut means slow conversion of thyroid hormones. Detoxify to keep these organs in top shape.

f. Manage stress and adrenal fatigue

Thyroid and adrenal function are closely linked. Managing thyroid means managing adrenals. Stress fires up the adrenals and cause adrenal fatigue. This will cause thyroid function to slow down. De-stress to reduce strain on the adrenals and also ease up on the thyroid.

g. Goitrous foods

Goiter slows down the function of the thyroid gland. Goitrogenic food can worsen goiter, which can cause hypothyroidism. Avoid goitrous foods like Brussels, sprouts, bok choy, cauliflower, mustard greens, broccoli, and other cruciferous vegetables. Also, avoid soy, tofu and lecithin.

II. Consume more foods that promote healing thyroid

a. Foods that are paced with macro- and micro-nutrients

Choose organic, hormone-free foods. The growth hormones fed to meats and poultry can interrupt the normal function of the endocrine system.

b. Protein and fat

Proteins and fats are the backbones of the body's hormones. Eat them in the right proportions and from the right sources. Choose healthy fat sources such as fish and seafood oil, olive oil and coconut oil. Also, eat foods that are naturally rich in healthy fats such as avocados and coconuts. Good protein sources are from lean cuts of meats, poultry without the skin on and from beans.

    c. Probiotics

Probiotics help restore the balance of good bacteria in the gut. Good bacteria help in preventing the absorption of bad compounds and toxins from the gut and into the blood. Add probiotics to the diet by eating foods that have naturally fermented. Examples are:

- Kim chee (Korean fermented veggies)
- Sauerkraut (not fermented in vinegar)
- Yoghurt
- Kombucha tea
- Kefir
- Coconut water
- Vegetable medley (fermented)

    d. Herbs and supplements

Get the recommended daily dose of vitamins and minerals such as vitamin D, calcium and selenium.

    e. Meditation
    f. Exercise

Exercise helps to restart the hormone balance. It also helps in better circulation of hormones and better cellular response.

III.   Balance according to the body's needs

Everyone has unique health needs. Cater to the individual needs by taking into consideration all the individual's needs according to age, height, weight, activity and overall health condition.

Chapter 5 Thyroid Diet Food Guide

Certain foods contain compounds that can influence thyroid function. There are foods that can improve thyroid levels. Some foods interfere with thyroid function. People should learn what foods help thyroid in functioning normally and which foods to avoid that can interfere with the thyroid glands.

Foods to eat

Avocado and potato

These foods are rich in amino acid tyrosine. Studies have found that low tyrosine level is linked to hypothyroidism.

Artichokes

Artichokes have powerful detoxifying effect on the liver. Clear liver means better at producing proteins that can bind and carry thyroid hormones for circulation in the blood.

Sea vegetables

These are notoriously rich in iodine, which a main component of thyroid hormone synthesis. Good ones include arame, kombu, kelp, dulse and wakame.

Beans

Beans contain an abundance of iodine. Aside from this trace mineral, beans are also good sources of fiber. The fiber helps to relieve constipation that most people with hypothyroidism suffer from.

Foods rich in Iodine (good for hypothyroidism)

- Iodized Salt
- Seaweeds and Seafoods
- Celtic Sea Salt
- Salt Water Fish
- Nori Rolls
- Sushi

Foods rich in Selenium (good for hypothyroidism)

- Meat

- Salmon
- Chicken
- Tuna
- Brazil Nuts
- Whole Unrefined Grains
- Dairy Products
- Onions
- Garlic

Herbs

Herbs help to boost the metabolism. Some help in detoxifying the body, such as cilantro, which removes mercury that is toxic to the thyroid gland.

- Black Pepper
- Tumeric
- Chilies
- Ginger
- Garlic
- Cinnamon
- Peppermint
- Parsley
- Cilantro
- Rosemary

Fruits

Fruits contain trace minerals such as iodine and selenium. They also contain antioxidants that detoxify the body and boost overall bodily function.

Cranberries, in particular, are rich in iodine. About 400 mcg (micrograms) of iodine is contained in ½ cup of this fruit.

Other thyroid-friendly fruits are:

- Apples

ESSENTIAL OILS BOX SET #16: Thyroid Diet & The Hypothyroidism Handbook

- Apricots
- Bananas
- Blueberries
- Blackberries
- Cherries
- Cranberries
- Dates
- Grapefruit
- Kiwi
- Papaya
- Pineapple
- Prunes
- Raspberries

Grains

Grains help to regulate sugar levels that can otherwise put off sugar balance. Good grains include:

- Amaranth
- Quinoa
- Buckwheat
- Brown Rice
- Wild Rice

Oils

Good oils are great fat sources, which the thyroid can use to synthesize thyroid hormones. Coconut oil, in particular, stimulates the thyroid gland to increase hormone production. Olive oil and raw butter also have good effects on thyroid function.

Foods to avoid (which can worsen hypothyroidism)

While foods can help stimulate better thyroid function, some foods have known negative effects on this gland. Avoid the following, which are detrimental to thyroid health:

- Cassava
- Kohlrabi
- Linseed
- Turnips
- Kale
- Peanuts
- Mustard
- Mustard Greens
- Cauliflower
- Millet
- Rutabagas
- Spinach
- Peaches
- Coffee

Goitrogenic foods

- Soybeans and related products
- Bamboo shoots
- Canola Oil
- Bok Choy
- Horseradish
- Sweet Potato
- Foods with Gluten
- Tempeh
- Garden Kres

ESSENTIAL OILS BOX SET #16: Thyroid Diet & The Hypothyroidism Handbook

- Babassu

Goitrogenic Chemicals

- Lithium
- Amiodarone
- Carbamazepine
- Oxazolidines
- Minocycline (MN)
- Iopanoic acid
- Thioureylene
- Propylthiouracil
- Sulfadimethoxine
- Phenobarbitone

Chapter 6 Thyroid Diet for Weight Loss

As has been previously mentioned, people can use the thyroid diet for weight loss. People suffering from hypothyroidism are the main reasons for this weight loss diet. Hypothyroidism can cause weight gain. In order to lose weight or at least maintain it at a normal level, experts advise using the specially formulated thyroid diet.

The most effective weight loss program designed for thyroid patients focuses not only on calorie counts but also on spacing caloric intake throughout the day. That is, the calculated calorie intake is taken in several mini-meals.

Also, experts believe that people who suffer from hypothyroidism need to adjust the proportions and distribution of macronutrient intake. That is, a meal should comprise of 40% proteins, 35% carbohydrates (from low glycemic index foods), and 25% fats, with 250 to 300 calories at each meal.

Let's take a closer look into the previous example:

A person who weighs 75 kilograms (165 pounds) with a thyroid condition (e.g., hypothyroidism) wants to lose weight safely.

Get the daily calorie needs: 75 kilograms X 25 = 1875 calories per day

Subtract 200 calories (thyroid factor, to account for thyroid condition):

    1875-200= 1675 calories per day for safe weight loss

Divide a day's worth of meals into mini-meals, with 300 calories each meal. To get the number of 300-calorie meals per day, divide the calorie for weight loss by 300:

    1675 calories / 300 = 5.58 or 6 mini-meals a day

This means that a person who weighs 75 kilograms would need to eat 6 mini meals each day, at 300 calories per meal in order to lose weight safely. The mini-meals should be evenly spaced out throughout the day.

The recommended rate of weight loss is at 1 kilogram or 2.2 pounds a week only. Going more than that can trigger starvation mode in the body. While the body still has adequate fat and energy stores, abruptly and severely reducing food intake will cause the body to recognize it as going into starvation. Instead of losing weight and burning fats, the body tries really hard to retain all the fats and to keep eating. Cravings will o over the top in this case, which can lead to serious overeating and gaining back more weight than what was initially lost.

So, in order to lose weight effectively and sustainably, lose weight gradually and safely.

Conclusion

Thank you again for purchasing this book!

I hope this book was able to help you to learn more about the thyroid gland, the disorders, and how these can be managed. The thyroid diet is an affective diet both for restoring thyroid health and in losing weight.

The next step is to start making that healthier choice. Start making the changes today and live a healthier life. The changes may be difficult at first but with solid determination to become a healthier person, it will all be worth it. Also, share with family and friends about this wonderful book and the knowledge it imparts. Get them to accompany you in this health journey and experience the health benefits of the thyroid diet.

Finally, if you enjoyed this book, please take the time to share your thoughts and post a review on Amazon. We do our best to reach out to readers and provide the best value we can. Your positive review will help us achieve that. It'd be greatly appreciated!

Thank you and good luck!

Book 2:
The Hypothyroidism Handbook:
BY LINDSEY P

An Everyday Guide to Natural Solutions of living with Hypothyroidism including increased energy, lasting weight loss, and general well-being

ESSENTIAL OILS BOX SET #16: Thyroid Diet & The Hypothyroidism Handbook

Copyright 2014 by Lindsey P - All rights reserved.

In no way is it legal to reproduce, duplicate, or transmit any part of this document in either electronic means or in printed format. Recording of this publication is strictly prohibited and any storage of this document is not allowed unless with written permission from the publisher. All rights reserved.

ESSENTIAL OILS BOX SET #16: Thyroid Diet & The Hypothyroidism Handbook

Table of Contents

Introduction 29

Chapter 1: Causes, Signs and Symptoms of Hypothyroidism 30

Chapter 2: Go Gluten Free! 33

Chapter 3: Eat your way to being healthy 35

Chapter 4: Vitamins, Minerals, and Nutrients 39

Chapter 5: Thyroid Stimulating Exercises 42

Chapter 6: Other Reminders 44

Conclusion 46

Check Out My Other Books 47

ESSENTIAL OILS BOX SET #16: Thyroid Diet & The Hypothyroidism Handbook

Introduction

I want to thank you and congratulate you for purchasing the book, "The Hypothyroidism Handbook: An Everyday Guide to Natural solutions of living with Hypothyroidism including increased energy, lasting weight loss and general well-being".

This book contains proven steps and strategies on how to treat Hypothyroidism naturally. Hypothyroidism is known as the condition where in one has an abnormally low production of thyroid hormones. Lacks of thyroid hormones affect the body in many ways, such as:

- An enlarged heart
- Having a hard time losing weight which leads to too much weight gain
- Worsening heart failure
- Accumulation of fluid in the lungs which can lead to many respiratory diseases

With the help of this book, you will get to know the signs and symptoms of Hypothyroidism, its causes, and the various natural ways that you can combat the disease. If you want to live a long and healthy life without Hypothyroidism, you have to start reading this book now.

Thanks again for purchasing this book, I hope you enjoy it!

Chapter 1: Causes, Signs and Symptoms of Hypothyroidism

Before you get to know what could be done to fight off the disease, you should first get to know what causes it in the first place. Listed below are the most common causes of Hypothyroidism:

- **Pregnancy.** When women are pregnant or in that span of time just after giving birth, they tend to produce antibodies courtesy of their thyroid glands and that's why thyroid hormone production is lessened. The rise of blood pressure while pregnant may cause a miscarriage to happen or may affect the fetus.

- **Autoimmune Diseases.** Those who suffer from autoimmune diseases such as Hashimoto's Thyroditis are more likely to develop Hypothyroidism as their immune system is not working properly to protect them.

- **Radiation Therapy.** If you are already suffering from cancers of the neck and head that require radiation to be treated, you may also get to suffer from Hypothyroidism in the future.

- **Thyroid Surgery.** Of course, surgeries involving the thyroid can be big causes of Hypothyroidism because it halts or diminishes Thyroid Production.

- **Medication.** There are certain types of medicine that causes Hypothyroidism, especially those that are used to treat Psychiatric diseases such as Lithium. It would be best for you to ask your doctor about the certain effects of the medicines that you are taking to your body.

- **Pituitary Disorder.** Sometimes, the Pituitary gland fails to produce the enough number of Thyroid Stimulating Hormones or TSH because there are benign tumors in the Pituitary Gland. These then cause Hypothyroidism to happen.

- **Congenital Diseases.** Some babies are born with defective thyroid glands or no thyroid glands at all. It may be a cause of problems during pregnancy or because their parents also have Hypothyroidism.

- **Iodine Deficiency.** You know why they say that you have to eat foods that are rich in Iodine? Well, it's because Iodine Deficiency causes a lot of diseases such as Goiter and in this case, Hypothyroidism.

Common Symptoms of Hypothyroidism:

ESSENTIAL OILS BOX SET #16: Thyroid Diet & The Hypothyroidism Handbook

Be aware and see if you are suffering from Hypothyroidism. If you are experiencing some of the symptoms listed below, you probably are.

- Dry skin
- Constipation
- An increased insensitivity to coldness
- Having a puffy face
- Unexplained weight gain
- Weak muscles
- Hoarseness
- Feeling over-fatigued or exhausted most of the time
- Swelling of the joints, pain and stiffness
- Irregular menstrual periods
- Heavy menstrual periods
- Tenderness and stiffness of the muscles
- Impaired memory
- An unusual thinning of the hair
- Depression
- Slow heart rate
- Heightened blood cholesterol level

In infants, you have to be wary of the following:

- Frequent choking
- Yellowing of the white part of the eyes and of the skin, as well. This condition is also called Jaundice and happens when an infant's liver cannot metabolize Bilirubin, a substance that causes red blood cells to be damaged.
- A puffy face
- A protruding and large tongue

- Sleeplessness
- Constipation

And as for children and teens:
- Late development of permanent teeth
- Poor mental development
- Delayed growth, which often results to a short stature
- Delayed puberty or onset of menstruation for teenage girls

Take note that once Hypothyroidism is not treated early, it may worsen and that's why as early as now, you have to make sure that you keep yourself safe from the worsening of this disease. Turn to the next chapter and get to learn about the various ways of combating Hypothyroidism.

Chapter 2: Go Gluten Free!

A Gluten-free diet is said to be the most effective, natural way of getting rid of Hypothyroidism. This is a kind of diet that excludes the Protein Gluten from one's daily meals. This is because Gluten is said to be the cause of certain diseases such as Celiac Disease and is also known to damage one's intestines and thyroid glands.

A lot of people find it hard to just leave their old eating habits behind and switch to a Gluten-free kind of life. There's also the thought that one may not get all the nutrients that one's body needs and that are essential to one's growth, such as Iron and Calcium, but Gluten Diet practitioners say that the diet really has done wonders for them and that it can easily help someone to get healthier and be able to fight many diseases such as Hypothyroidism.

Which foods are allowed in this diet?

- Fresh eggs
- Unprocessed seeds, nuts and beans
- Fruits and vegetables
- Dairy products
- Fresh poultry, fish and meat which are not battered, marinated or coated
- Grains such as Buckwheat, Arrowroot, Flax, Corn, Cornmeal, Amaranth, Rice, Millet, Quinoa, Soy, Sorghum, Teff and Tapioca

Which foods should you avoid?

- Wheat
- Rye
- Barley, which means that you should also avoid beer, malt vinegar and malt flavoring that are made from Barley
- Triticale, a mix of wheat and rye
- Durum Flour
- Kamut
- Semolina
- Bulgur

- Farina
- Graham Flour
- Spelt

Aside from these, you should also avoid the foods listed below unless they are labeled as "Gluten-free":

- Pasta
- French Fries
- Gravy
- Candies, cookies and crackers
- Cereals
- Bread
- Salad dressings
- Seasoned potato chips and tortilla chips
- Seasoned rice mixes
- Soy sauce and other sauces
- Vegetables with sauce
- Self-basting poultry
- Processed or canned food such as Luncheon Meat and Corned Beef
- Soup bases and soup

With the right amount of discipline and self-control, you surely will be able to adhere to the Gluten Diet and allow yourself to live a longer and happier life. In the next chapter, you will learn about more ways of letting go of Hypothyroidism by means of what you eat.

ESSENTIAL OILS BOX SET #16: Thyroid Diet & The Hypothyroidism Handbook

Chapter 3: Eat your way to being healthy

If you cannot let go of your old eating habits and switch to the Gluten Diet easily, don't worry because you would still be able to combat the disease. You just have to be aware of what you eat and learn how to eat only nutritious kinds of food.

But what foods can help you in getting rid of Hypothyroidism? And what should you avoid? Here's what you need to know.

Get rid or eliminate coffee, sugar and carbohydrates

Eat non-starchy foods and vegetables, instead so that your body would be cleansed well and would not rely on sugar to live. Too much Sugar may also cause Hypothyroidism and other diseases such as Diabetes. Your body treats Carbohydrates like sugar and that's why you have to lessen your intake.

Fat can be your friend

Fat is considered as the great balancer of hormonal pathways—which means that you need to have them in your life. After all, if you are going to exercise after consuming some fat, you would be able to burn them away and still be in the right state of your body and in the target weight that you want to be in. You could get healthy fats from avocados, fish, nut butters, nuts, flax, Olive Oil, Ghee, full fat cheese, cottage cheese, yogurt and products made out of coconut milk.

Add Protein in your System

While Gluten is not allowed when it comes to beating Hypothyroidism, other kinds of Proteins are actually recommended for you. Right kinds of protein can be found in whole and grass-fed eggs, fresh fish, grass-fed meats, quinoa, nuts, and nut butters, as well.

Glutathione

More than the number of beauty products filled with Glutathione that have sprouted in the market like mushrooms, Glutathione is actually a healthy anti-oxidant that can be produced by the body by consuming certain kinds of food products, such as: raw eggs, avocados, garlic, squash, spinach, peaches, asparagus, broccoli, and grapefruit. Glutathione helps in producing thyroid hormones and protecting and healing thyroid glands. However, you should also take note that you have to control yourself from eating too much of some of them because they contain Goitrogens, which may interfere with the way your thyroid works. Foods rich in Goitrogen that must be lessened from your diet include:

Kale

- Rutabaga

- Broccoli
- Cauliflower
- Brussels Sprouts
- Millet
- Spinach
- Turnips
- Watercress
- Strawberries
- Peaches
- Peanuts
- Soybeans
- Radish

Take everything in moderation. Don't worry though because you do not have to completely eliminate them from your diet. Once cooked, these food products lose goitrogens. You just have to be careful about eating them raw and in large amounts.

Iodine

As mentioned earlier, Iodine is very important in keeping the body healthy and making sure that you are able to combat Hypothyroidism. It is also great in the prevention of diseases like cretinism, goiter, and mental disabilities, and also aids in the lessening of fatigue, lethargy, weight gain and depression. Iodine is essential in the production of thyroid hormones and that's why you have to include it in your diet. Aside from Iodized salt, which has been proven to reduce the number of patients affected with Hypothyroidism in the United States, other food products that are rich in Iodine include: Dried Seaweed, cod fish, unpeeled baked potato, fish sticks, shrimp, milk, canned tuna with oil, boiled egg, cooked navy beans and cooked turkey breast, as well.

Get rid of Inflammatory Foods

Inflammatory foods, or those that cause inflammation inside the body are a big no-no when it comes to fighting Hypothyroidism. People do not usually know which kinds of foods are considered inflammatory and that's why it is very important to check food labels in order for you to understand what it is that you will be eating. Inflammatory foods include:

ESSENTIAL OILS BOX SET #16: Thyroid Diet & The Hypothyroidism Handbook

- **Those with High Trans Fat.** Again, you have to check food labels for this. Trans fat is very inflammable and damages the cells that line your blood vessels which makes it very dangerous.

- **Cheeseburgers.** While they may be delicious and are great comfort foods, research has it that high amount of animal fat causes inflammation. Aside from that, cheeseburgers also cause tissue and gland damage—which might lead to Hypothyroidism instead of getting rid of it.

- **Sugar.** The body cannot break down each and every bit of sugar that you intake and that's why it is essential that you lessen the amount of sugar in your diet.

- **White bread.** This instantly breaks down to sugar as it is full of carbohydrates and as mentioned earlier, you do not need a lot of carbohydrates if you are trying to take care of yourself and trying to get rid of hypothyroidism. White bread makes the body more inflammable and that's not what you'd want to happen.

- **Alcohol.** Aside from the fact that beer is usually made from Barley, too much alcohol makes it easier for bacteria to make their way through your system and damage different tissues and organs. Alcohol also leads to inflammation—you've probably noticed this by the burning sensation you feel while drinking alcohol and just dismissed it as nothing, when in fact, it already damages your system.

- **Omega 6 Fatty Acids.** The difference of these from the healthy Omega 3 Fatty Acids is that they do not do the body good. Omega-6 rich foods include walnuts, vegetable oils and heavy seeds.

- **MSG.** You probably already know that MSG is bad for you and that's why you should cut back on junk foods. MSG can cause a lot of inflammation and may also cause diseases, especially thyroid and kidney related ones and that's why you should cut back on it.

- **Too much milk.** Again, you have to take everything in moderation because too much of anything is never a good thing. Don't drink too much milk especially if you are lactose-intolerant because you will not be able to digest it well.

Detoxify

Going on Detox is not just for those who are trying to get a great figure or are trying to diet just to look good. Detoxification is important for your body and mind to be rejuvenated and refreshed once again. There are so many juice cleanses available right now that you can choose from, or you can choose to make your own if that's more your thing. A combination of Chlorella, Turmeric, Cilantro and Milk Thistle is said to be the best kind of juice cleanse mix that you can take in order to detoxify. You can also juice your choice of fruits and vegetables—what matters is that you drink them for them to work.

Keep these things in mind the next time you go grocery shopping or the next time you eat at a brand new restaurant. Your health should always be your top priority.

ESSENTIAL OILS BOX SET #16: Thyroid Diet & The Hypothyroidism Handbook

Chapter 4: Vitamins, Minerals, and Nutrients

Aside from eating the right kind of food, it is also very important for you to take the right kind of supplements and get the best nutrients for you to be able to fight Hypothyroidism well. Here are what you should intake, some foods included, and what you should avoid in order to be able to take care of your thyroid glands better and in order for your body to produce more thyroid hormones:

Stay away from BPA

BPA or Bisphenol A is commonly found in plastic bottles—the kind where you drink juices or teas or even water from. BPA damages your endocrine system and therefore, have bad effects on your thyroid. So, the next time you get thirsty, make it a point to drink only from glass or stainless steel cans. Also, look for the "BPA Free" sign from those plastic bottles to ensure that they are safe to use and drink from.

A Daptogen Supplements

A Daptogen Supplements are known to lower cortisol levels which in turn makes it easy for your thyroid glands to produce more thyroid hormones for you. You need A Daptogen to get rid of Adrenal Fatigue which is also one of the causes of Hypothyroidism. Tulasi, an herb cultivated for medicinal purposes which is also known as Holy Basil, and Ashwagandha or Winter Cherry are great sources of A Daptogen. As these herbs are more commonly found in India than in other parts of the world, taking supplements made out of them would be better than scouring the world to take hold of the herbs yourself.

A need for Selenium

Selenium, although not a very popular mineral, is actually important because it plays a key role in making metabolism faster. Once your metabolism is fast, it means that your body will be able to digest what you have been eating. This way, you're being able to combat Hypothyroidism. Aside from that, it is also known to battle other diseases such as Lung Cancer, Crohn's Disease and Prostate Cancer, as well.

Great sources of Selenium include: Grains, Poultry, Beef, Nuts, Brazil Nuts, Tuna, Herring, Red Snapper and Cod. Whole foods are also good sources of Selenium as the mineral gets dissolved once processing takes place.

Vitamin D

A walk in the sun before 10 am would be good to give your body the amount of Vitamin D that it needs to combat certain kinds of Cancer and Hypothyroidism, as well. Vitamin D3 supplements are also good to give you the Vitamin D that you lack in your system as lack of Vitamin D causes your glands not to produce thyroid hormones that are essential for you.

Iron

Iron is not only good for those who are suffering from Anemia, but is also good for your thyroid glands to produce more thyroid hormones that will help you become strong and will help you say goodbye to Hypothyroidism for good. Aside from taking Iron supplements, you may also eat foods that are rich in Iron, such as egg yolks, red meat, raisins, prunes, spinach, collards, beans, chick peas, lentils, soybeans, artichokes, liver, chicken giblets and turkey, as well. Take Iron along with Vitamin C and you surely will be able to combat the disease even better as Vitamin C is good against inflammation.

Probiotics

Probiotics are more commonly known as good bacteria. Your body needs these as they are the ones who get to fight bad bacteria from taking over your body. Good sources of Probiotics include:

- **Yogurt.** Yogurt is considered as the best source of Probiotics and is also considered as the best substitute for ice cream. Lactobacillus Shirota Strain-filled yogurt products are what you should go for. Aside from being good against Hypothyroidism, yogurt is also good for lessening gas, diarrhea and other kinds of digestive problems.

- **Kefir.** Kefir is a probiotic-filled drink that is said to have originated from Caucasus Mountains of Eurasia. It's almost the same as yogurt but is bubbly, creamy and thick and is good in battling yeast infections.

- **Milk with Probiotics.** There are some milk products that are made with probiotics. You'll know that they are if they are greenish in color and are creamier than your usual kind of milk. It is also commonly known as sweet acidophilus milk. Buttermilk is also known to be rich in probiotics so you can try that, as well.

- **Miso Soup.** Miso is quite popular in Japan and other parts of Asia as a soup made with fish and mustard plus the vegetable bok choi. A bowl of Miso soup contains at least 160 bacteria strains which are about the proper amount that you need each day. It is also low in calories and carbohydrates which make it perfect for someone who is trying to get rid of Hypothyroidism.

- **Sauerkraut.** These days, Sauerkraut is mainly used for sausage dishes and that's why you would not have a hard time trying to find it. Go for unpasteurized Sauerkraut because pasteurization is known to kill good bacteria.

- **Soft Cheese.** Gouda and other kinds of fermented cheese are able to survive in your system for a long time. This means that you will be safe from bad bacteria that damages cells and glands and so you will be able to eliminate the sources of Hypothyroidism.
- **Sourdough Bread.** Sourdough bread is popular for being great in making digestion and metabolism faster. It is also full of Lactobacilli, which are great examples of good bacteria.
- **Sour Pickles.** Pickles are also a good source of probiotics. Go for those that are naturally fermented or those that do not use vinegar in the fermentation process. These pickles also gave metabolic and digestive properties that are truly good for you.
- **Tempeh.** Tempeh is a popular kind of Indonesian Patty that is rich in natural antibiotics that fight bacteria and is also very high in protein. You would not have a hard time liking Tempeh because it is deliciously nutty and smoky and may also taste like a mushroom. You can also marinate Tempeh and add it to other dishes and recipes.
- **Or, you can just try taking Probiotic Supplements.** They are available in liquid, tablet or capsule form and will give you the right amount of Probiotics that you need.

Chapter 5: Thyroid Stimulating Exercises

Contrary to popular belief, there are actually some exercises that patients who suffer from Hypothyroidism can do. Just because you are suffering from Hypothyroidism does not mean that you can no longer workout or use your body for physical activities. Thinking this way would just worsen your disease.

Walking Daily

You'd be surprised to know how much walking contributes to your well-being. If you need to go somewhere and it's not far away from home, why not try walking instead of taking a can or riding other forms of public transport? Aside from the fact that you will be able to save some money, walking is simple and will also help you appreciate the beauty of your surroundings even better. Walking for around 20 to 40 minutes per day is already good to combat Hypothyroidism—it helps you lose weight and makes your metabolism faster. It also lets your thyroid glands work at an optimal rate.

Jogging

You don't need to do it professionally. Do it early in the morning or at night, upon coming home. You can do it in your own backyard if you want or use your village or the nearby park to jog. What's important is that you do it once or twice a week so that you'd get to burn all the extra fats that you have accumulated and so that your body will feel refreshed.

Circuit Training

Circuit Training is also proven to help reduce the risk of Hypothyroidism. Circuit Training also helps lower insulin levels, which in turn protects you against Diabetes. Some examples of these exercises include push-ups, lunges, curl-ups, bench presses, and sit ups for a couple of repetitions. If you do not like to go to the gym, then you can also do the exercises at the comforts of your own home. Rest a bit to catch your breath then do them again. You can devote at least 10 to 20 minutes of your day to Circuit Training and you will be alright.

Get to know your Acupressure Points

Devoting a bit of your time to massage or relax different Acupressure Points in your body would do wonders for your system when it comes to battling Hypothyroidism. You can do these for at least 2 to 5 times daily for them to work better. Some examples include:

- **Neck-Press.** Sit down and close your eyes and interlace your hands behind your neck, or on your nape. Bow your head down a bit and just relax. This way, you will be able to stretch your neck muscles. Then, bring your elbows together in front of you and compress the sides of your neck using your hands. Raise your head as you stretch gently and inhale and exhale as you relax. Repeat the exercise for at least 2 minutes.

- **K 27.** K 27 is known as both sides of your sternum. Just take long, deep breaths and turn your head from side to side. Allow yourself to feel how your neck region relaxes and just go and breathe deeply as you hold the K27 spots. Tilt your head up as you inhale, and down as you exhale and visualize the things that you want to have or the things you want to do someday. This is a good way of meditating, as well so not only do you help your body, you also get to clear your mind of its worries.
- **Temples.** Use your index and middle finger to massage your temples. Sit down, relax and massage both temples in circular motions. These will easily help you ease the pain that you are feeling and would also help you relax.

Chapter 6: Other Reminders

Aside from what was discussed in earlier chapters, here are some of the other things that you should keep in mind for you to be able to battle your disease.

Eliminate Stress

Stress causes you to feel bad about yourself, does not put your mind at ease, and also is one of the reasons why you get to suffer from some diseases such as Hypothyroidism because it causes your adrenal and thyroid glands to be exhausted. In order to eliminate stress, you should:

- **Try Meditation**. Go to a quiet place, think of a mantra, repeat it over and over again, and then make sure that you get to understand that it is true. For example, say "I can do this" or "I can get rid of this disease", and believe in it for it to be true. The power of positive thinking would really do you wonders so do not underestimate it.

- **Get an ample amount of sleep**. Sleeping for 6 to 8 hours each night, even if you are already an adult, is essential to help you become healthy and in top shape. If you get the right amount of sleep, you'd feel better about yourself and about the day that you are going to embark on. Getting the right amount of sleep equals happiness, so why would you deprive yourself of sleep?

- **Write your feelings down.** Creating a blog or writing on a journal always helps to make you feel better about yourself because you will be able to put your feelings out and let go of whatever it is that's bothering you. This way, you will be able to understand yourself better and get a clear mind when it comes to knowing that you will be able to battle the disease and let go of it—just as long as you believe that you can.

- **Do what you love.** It's much like a cliché, but doing what you love can do you wonders. When you know that you are doing things that people say you cannot do, or that are deemed as stupid, even if they are not, would surely make you feel better about yourself and would help lessen the stress in your life.

Drink lots of water

Another fact of life that most people take for granted is the fact that water is important to good health. It is also a given fact that drinking water is essential for those who have thyroid problems or thyroid related diseases. Aside from the traditional 8 glasses a day, you'd have to drink another glass for each pound that you want to lose.

Drink Green Tea

Research has it that aside from being able to cleanse your system, Green Tea is also good in making you more adept in exercising and in helping you feel better about yourself while exercising. And, it also calms you down which makes you feel less stressed and more motivated.

Remove Silver Fillings

If you've gotten treatment or Pasta for your teeth, you may have gotten silver fillings without being aware of it. These are also called Amalgam Fillings and may have high amounts of mercury which are dangerous to the body. It would be good to ask your dentist about what's in your Pasta before getting one, and if you already have one, then look for a dentist that offers Amalgam-free types of Pasta so that you will be safer. Amalgam also disrupts thyroid production and that's why you have to get rid of it.

And, Try Heat Therapy

Going to the sauna, taking a hot shower, or relaxing in a hot spring is great not only because they are able to help you relax and feel calmer, they are also able to eliminate stored toxins. It's important to get rid of the body's stored toxins as these only blocks the production of thyroid hormones which then causes Hypothyroidism.

Conclusion

Thank you again for purchasing this book!

I hope this book was able to help you to understand what Hypothyroidism is all about, how you will know that you have the disease and what to do to get rid of it.

The next step is to not only read and keep this book, but to actually try what is written in here. If you want to let go of your disease, then you should believe that you can and you should do whatever you can to let go of it and not let it take over your life. With the help of this book, you certainly can do it.

Finally, if you enjoyed this book, please take the time to share your thoughts and post a review on Amazon. We do our best to reach out to readers and provide the best value we can. Your positive review will help us achieve that. It'd be greatly appreciated!

Thank you and good luck!

ESSENTIAL OILS BOX SET #16: Thyroid Diet & The Hypothyroidism Handbook

Check Out My Other Books

Below you'll find some of my other popular books that are popular on Amazon and Kindle as well. Simply click on the links below to check them out. Alternatively, you can visit my author page on Amazon to see other work done by me.

Coconut Oil for Easy Weight Loss

http://amzn.to/1i5f45p

Carrier Oils For Beginners

http://amzn.to/1sbqUQP

Natural Homemade Cleaning Recipes For Beginners

http://amzn.to/1izDB2m

Essential Oils & Aromatherapy

http://amzn.to/1ouuZTx

Superfoods that Kickstart Your Weight Loss

http://amzn.to/1eyHdku

The Best Secrets Of Natural Remedies

http://amzn.to/1gmHd7y

The Hyperthyroidism Handbook

http://amzn.to/1kqLQCp

ESSENTIAL OILS BOX SET #16: Thyroid Diet & The Hypothyroidism Handbook

Essential Oils & Weight Loss For Beginners
http://amzn.to/Q83bFp

Top Essential Oil Recipes
http://amzn.to/1lSrhSC

Soap Making For Beginners
http://amzn.to/1fkmYwr

Body Butters For Beginners
http://amzn.to/1fWjwJe

Apple Cider Vinegar For Beginners
http://amzn.to/1joDzX2

Homemade Body Scrubs & Masks For Beginners
http://amzn.to/1jjLRIO

The Beginners Guide To Medicinal Plants
http://amzn.to/1vSujr6

The Beginners Guide To Making Your Own Essential Oils
http://amzn.to/1piUNSB

The Beginners Alkaline Miracle Diet
http://amzn.to/1sDVaVE

ESSENTIAL OILS BOX SET #16: Thyroid Diet & The Hypothyroidism Handbook

Thyroid Diet

http://amzn.to/1piW2RY

Essential Oils Box Set #1 (Weight Loss + Essential Oil Recipes

http://amzn.to/1qlYWWP

Essential Oils Box Set #2 (Weight Loss + Essential Oil & Aromatherapy

http://amzn.to/1qlYWWP

Essential Oils Box Set #3 Coconut Oil + Apple Cider Vinegar

http://amzn.to/1oIFZJw

Essential Oils Box Set #4 Body Butters & Top Essential Oil Recipes

http://amzn.to/1jSxURJ

Essential Oils Box Set #5 Soap Making & Homemade Body Scrubs

http://amzn.to/RAvJYo

Essential Oils Box Set #6 Body Butters & Body Scrubs

http://amzn.to/RAvSel

Essential Oils Box Set #7 Top Essential Oils & Best Kept Secrets Of Natural Remedies

http://amzn.to/1gvsRCq

Essential Oils Box Set #8 Homemade Cleaning Recipes & Essential Oil Recipes

http://amzn.to/1gxFAVb

ESSENTIAL OILS BOX SET #16: Thyroid Diet & The Hypothyroidism Handbook

Essential Oils Box Set #9 Essential Oil and Weight Loss & Carrier Oils

http://amzn.to/1jmcEPP

Essential Oils Box Set #10 Hyperthyroidism Manual & Hypothyroidism Manual

http://amzn.to/1nHgJU4

Essential Oils Box Set #11 Carrier Oils for Beginners & Coconut Oil for Easy Weight Loss

http://amzn.to/1nHfy6X

Essential Oils Box Set #12 Essential Oils Weight Loss & Essential Oils Aromatherapy & Natural Homemade Cleaning Supplies & Top Essential Oil Recipes & Carrier Oils

http://amzn.to/1nHfy6X

Essential Oils Box Set #13 Superfoods & Essential Weight Loss & Essential Aromatherapy & Body Butters & Soap Making

http://amzn.to/1nUds6v

Essential Oils Box Set #14 Weight Loss & Apple Cider Vinegar & Body Butters & Homemade Body Scrubs & Coconut Oil for Beginners

http://amzn.to/1i1qYOd

Essential Oils Box Set #15 The Beginners Guide To Making your Own Essential Oils & The Beginners Guide to Medicinal Plants

http://amzn.to/1m6wNC4

Essential Oils Box Set #16 Thyroid Diet & Hypothyroidism Handbook

http://amzn.to/1wmtIOI

ESSENTIAL OILS BOX SET #16: Thyroid Diet & The Hypothyroidism Handbook

Essential Oils Box Set #17 Top Essential Oil Recipes & The Beginners Guide to Making Your Own Essential Oils
http://amzn.to/1BGYhBu

If the links do not work, for whatever reason, you can simply search for these titles on the Amazon website to find them.

www.ingramcontent.com/pod-product-compliance
Lightning Source LLC
Chambersburg PA
CBHW071826170526
45167CB00003B/1440